THE POWER OF NUTRITION

A Dietary Approach and Comprehensive Guide to Managing Eczema

JAMES HALEN

Contents

INTRODUCTION

If we are to take review our anatomy lessons, the skin is identified as the largest organ of the human body. The adult human body contains an average of 14 to 18 square feet of skin. The skin is primarily responsible for providing protection, allowing sensation as well as secretion. It also assists in the regulation of the body's temperature.

Proper skin care is an integral part of our day to day health and wellness routine. In fact, there are some individuals, especially women, who have no qualms of going out of their way to nurture their skin through regular application of products formulated to maintain the elasticity and suppleness of the skin.

As a protective shield, the skin protects our bodies from mechanical impact such that of blow and pressure as well as thermal impact like cold and heat. However, aside from its important function, healthy, clear and glowing skin is one of the key indicators of good health. It also significantly contributes to the overall attractiveness of the person.

Unfortunately, not everyone is able to achieve and maintain healthy and good-looking skin. For some people who are afflicted with skin irritations and allergies, the constant need to hide angry welts, infected blisters, blotchy and mottled skin can be a curse. If the skin problem is a recurring one, it can considerably dent one's confidence and self-esteem, especially when dealing with people.

One of the most common types of skin problems that have afflicted millions of people across the globe, not sparing infants and seniors, is eczema.

For anyone who has dealt with or continue to suffer eczema, severe and chronic cases can easily become a debilitating condition. Eczema is a condition that is suffered by many and yet few people openly talk about it. It's embarrassing, restricting and overly discomforting to say the least.

With hundreds of "miracle cures" available in the market today, the search for a treatment that works can be an arduous, expensive, frustrating one. In fact, for some, it's a distressful, confusing and even a depressing experience. But don't lose hope just yet. This guide is specifically designed to address stubborn cases of eczema and eliminate the problem right down from its roots for good. It is possible to have clear, healthy looking skin.

And yes, within the next 14 days.

I too have suffered severe eczema since childhood. It is not a disease that you will want to wish on anyone. The sleepless nights, the endless scratching, the unpleasant sight of infected skin, the expensive treatments that only provide temporary relief – trust me, I am familiar with all those, and then some.

Over the years, I have dedicated myself into helping people survive and live life without eczema. It is possible. Let me help you write your very own success story in the battle with the dreaded, overly persistent eczema.

WHAT IS ECZEMA?

If you are suffering from mild, intense or recurring case of rashes or any form of skin irritation that triggers itchiness and redness of the skin, this may be symptoms of dermatitis.

Dermatitis is a medical term used to refer to a group of skin conditions that commonly exhibit a rash and often causes varying degrees of skin inflammation.

In general, these rashes are triggered by a certain type of allergic reaction, which can be categorized into different groups, based on what specific type of allergen has caused it. Among the best well known and widely common type of skin allergic reaction under this category is eczema or what is medically known as eczematous dermatitis.

HOW DO YOU KNOW IF YOU HAVE ECZEMA?

If you have a rash, whether is a mild case, a severe one, don't panic! Typically, rashes go away on its own. However, if you have eczema, the simple rash may go away at fits – but it tends to come back, again and again as a chronic skin condition.

It is important to note that not all rashes itch. However, in the case of eczema, you are most likely to experience intense itchiness, making it too difficult to tamp down the natural urge to scratch. In most cases, an irritation will start around the folds of your elbow's undersides or at the back portion of your knees. It can also appear on certain areas of the face or other parts of the body.

Since not all rashes can be categorized as eczema, it is generally best that you consult your doctor in order to fully determine what skin disorder you are suffering from and what is causing it.

In most cases, eczema appears like overly dry, cracked skin with a rough texture. In severe cases, it can be reddish in color and inflamed. It is also often itchy and irritating.

If you are not quite sure whether you have eczema or not, below are some symptoms that you can go through and check on yourself. Keep in mind that these symptoms are often recurring in nature. Among the most common symptoms include:

Dry and Exceedingly Itchy Skin. This is brought about by the fact that the skin is unable to give sufficient waterproofing, which then speeds up the evaporation process of natural moisture from the surface of the skin, leading to abnormal dryness. In cases of eczema, the itching is severe in nature, prompting you to constantly scratch the affected and surrounding areas. However, the more you succumb to the temptation of scratching the rashes, the more the itchiness is aggravated.

Blisters With Discharges and Crust Formation. If you are unable to stop scratching excessively, the rashes will develop into bright red blisters. When the eczema is active, the blisters are generally small, appearing along the exterior topmost layer of the skin, which tends to grow crusty over time.

Blisters usually split, which triggers the release of fluid secreted on the surface of the skin. When the secretion dries up, it typically develops into yellowish crusty scabs that stay on the skin for several days.

Inflammation of the skin. When the rashes worsens and becomes inflamed with some degree of swelling, it becomes irritated.

Bleeding. For severely irritated skin that has become inflamed, infected and raw, bleeding may also occur. This is mainly brought about by excessive scratching.

Leathery Skin. Extreme dryness of the skin can turn it into a somewhat leathery texture, with more or far lesser amount of pigment present compared to that of the normal, healthy skin. This condition is also called lichenification, which is characterized as the thickening of the skin, coupled with the exaggeration skin markings, giving it a rubbery, somewhat bark-like look. This again is brought about by excessive scratching. The pigmentation of this area of the skin differs from the normal tone because of the continuous itch-scratch cycle

Are you experiencing any of these common symptoms of eczema? What do you need to do? First, restrain the need to scratch the affected area as it can only aggravate the condition. You also need to keep your skin moisturized. Do not allow your skin to go dry.

In order to treat the condition, you need to determine the trigger that has caused the allergic reaction to address the root source of the problem. Then of course, you need to formulate the right treatment plan accordingly.

TYPES OF ECZEMA

According to the National Eczema Association, eczema refers to a broad term used to refer to any type or form of dermatitis, otherwise known as an itchy rash. This is a condition wherein the topmost skin layer becomes red, itchy, inflamed or dry.

If you believe you are suffering from eczema, it is generally best to have a full knowledge on what type of eczema it is in order to determine the appropriate treatment plan.

There are different types of eczema out there. In certain cases, a person can develop more than one type. To give you a clear idea on the most common types and how it looks like, below are the top five (5) types of eczema.

ATOPIC DERMATITIS (AD)

The atopic dermatitis type of eczema has been identified to be among the more severe and recurring (chronic) type of eczema. It is very alarming as it affects a large percentage of the human population.

Atopic dermatitis is characterized condition that triggers severe itchiness and inflammation skin. This condition can occur at any age and almost always begin during the childhood years, typically among babies or infants.

There is an estimated 65% of individuals suffering from eczema were diagnosed in their first few years from birth and 90% of them experienced it before the age five.

When children with atopic dermatitis gets older, this condition can more often improve or go away but for others who don't grow out of it, atopic dermatitis can be a life-long ordeal. A person with hay fever and asthma is more likely to develop this kind of skin disease, which is why atopic dermatitis is categorized as an "atopy" disease.

Causes: Atopic Dermatitis is the one of the most common forms of eczema. This skin condition is not infectious or contagious. A concrete conclusion on the underlying cause of atopic dermatitis remains unknown, although it is widely believed to be triggered by hereditary factors or is genetically acquired. Other possible causes include environmental factors such as the climate.

CONTACT DERMATITIS (ALLERGIC OR IRRITANT)

Contact dermatitis refers to a physiological response that can take place when the skin directly comes into contact with foreign materials or substances, which triggers a rash or irritation of the skin. Allergens or irritants are identified substances that can set off that burning sensation, along with itchiness and/or redness. There are basically two (2) different types of Contact Dermatitis, the Allergic Contact Dermatitis and the other is the Irritant Contact Dermatitis.

ALLERGIC CONTACT DERMATITIS

The first type is the Allergic Contact Dermatitis or more popularly referred to as ACD refers to the response by the immune system to an irritant substance in direct contact the skin. There are roughly several thousand different types of substances that can possibly trigger this allergic reaction. Among the widely common substances that are identified as irritants are largely found in certain plant life like the poison ivy. Others can be present in rubber, antibiotics, bottled perfumes and scents, preservatives, and some forms of metals. Even certain formulations of lotions and commercial creams and ointments that are used in the treatment of dermatitis can also pose as triggers of allergic reactions.

IRRITANT CONTACT DERMATITIS

The second one is the Irritant Contact Dermatitis on the other hand, is triggered by some chemical substance that causes damage afflicting directly the skin. Acids, products containing alkalis (certain drain cleaners), strong soaps, solvents (acetone used for nail polish removal), and plants (such as peppers and poinsettias) are among the typical examples of irritating substances that may damage skin.

Skin sensitivity may vary from one person to another. There are times that even mild soaps that are specifically formulated for sensitive skin and certain brands of detergents may cause irritation of some individuals after frequent and/or prolonged use or contact.

DYSHIDROTIC DERMATITIS

Another form of eczema is the Dyshidrotic Dermatitis also known as "Acute Vesiculobullous Hand Eczema" is a form of eczema, which is two times more common among women. This skin condition is characterized by small blisters visible in the hands and feet and is felt with itching and burning sensations.

This usually starts on the sides as itchy little bumps and then develops into a rash. People between the ages of 20 to 40 are the most common individuals to develop this form of eczema. Children can rarely have this but in most cases can be developed in children with atopic dermatitis.

Causes: Like atopic dermatitis, causes of it is still unknown but is strongly believed that environmental factors such as the weather and events occurring within the body (e.g., having another medical condition) can play a role.

NUMMULAR DERMATITIS

Nummular (meaning "coin-shaped") dermatitis is characterized by round-to oval shaped itchy lesions that can target any area of the human body but particularly affects the legs and buttocks area. One or many welts appear, and often persist for several weeks or even months.

This form of eczema is more common among males. Discoid eczema is not communicable or contagious to other people, although secondary infection can be triggered by bacteria. Eruptions of nummular dermatitis are often recurrent and chronic and appear at any age but usually in people in their 60's and is typically experienced in winter season.

Causes: Unfortunately there is no information to tell what causes it but is said to be worsened by stress and caffeine.

SEBORRHEIC DERMATITIS

Seborrheic Dermatitis, another common form of eczema is a form of skin condition that is characterized by flaky scales that range between whitish to yellowish in color. The most common areas affected are the oily areas of the body particularly the scalp area, creases of the nose, the eyelids and the eyebrows, the skin at the back of the ears as well as in the middle of the chest.

Seborrheic dermatitis appears to run in families. It affects an estimated 3% to 5% of the entire population, but is found to very more common among men, and is known to peak during the infancy stage as well as upon reaching middle age. Up to 85% of the people infected with the human immunodeficiency virus (HIV) have seborrheic dermatitis.

Causes: Despite various studies conducted, medical experts were unable to determine and identify the specific causes of this condition. However, the popular assumption is that it is brought about by the combination of excessive production of oil in the skin as well as the irritation triggered by yeast known as malessizia.

Also, factors such as stress, fatigue, oiliness of the skin, sporadic use of shampoos or infrequent skin cleaning, along with the usual use of cream or lotion that is formulated with alcohol, certain types of skin disorders like acne, as well as obesity. Other factors such as genetic, environmental, hormonal, and immune-system factors are also known to increase the risk of having this condition.

COMPREHENSIVE APPROACHES TO ECZEMA

Once you have fully determined the type of eczema you have, it can focus your efforts on knowing how to best handle and treat the condition. While all these different types are generally known as a form of eczema, each condition requires distinct approaches when it comes to skin care and treatment.

ATOPIC DERMATITIS

At present, there is still no available cure to get rid of atopic dermatitis. However, this does not mean you cannot manage the symptoms. There are a number of treatments that you can use to sooth and relieve the skin irritation as well as keep tightly in check and control possible outbreak.

A doctor makes the diagnosis based on the typical pattern of the rash and often on whether other family members have allergies. Also management chosen by the doctor for the patient relies on the extent and length of the eczema. No cure exists, but itching can be relieved with the following:

TOPICAL TREATMENTS

Topical drugs such as ointments, creams or lotions are the most commonly used treatment of people with this form of eczema. When the surface of the skin is irritated, raw or cracked, many of the topical products may sting or burn during the first application. This sensitive reaction will gradually diminish as the eczema condition improves. Here are the topical drugs that could be applied:

EMOLLIENTS. Emollients are formulated to supply additional moisture to the skin as well as aid in the prevention of further water loss. Emollients are considered to be among the most important component of eczema management and treatment. The use of lipid-containing emollients considerably decreases inflammation and concomitant oxidative stress in adult patients with mild-to-moderate atopic dermatitis.

Finding the ideal emollient that will work best for you can turn out to be a case of trial and error. Costly emollients can't be more effective than the more inexpensive ones because they more often than not contain perfume or other ingredients that can irritate the skin.

It is generally advised that emollients are used at least two times a day all over the skin. For best results, the treatment should be applied to the affected area within the first 3 minutes after a bath or shower in order to fully maximize its ability to retain moisture.

To date, there is no evidence that emollients improve atopic dermatitis directly. However, emollients are widely used because they improve the appearance and symptoms of the dry skin associated with this condition.

TOPICAL STEROIDS. Another effective treatment are topical steroids are considered to be a staple in the treatment for mild degree to moderate cases of eczema. Topical steroids are also used as a form of treatment for severe atopic dermatitis and as a way to help gradually reduce the dosage as well as the dependency to oral medications and the need for ultraviolet light. When it is used correctly, topical steroids are also very effective, most particularly in the treatment of flare-ups of eczema. They help keep down the inflammation and itching.

Application of this type of medication to the affected skin of a person with atopic eczema should not to be more than twice a day. One cannot benefit or increase the potency of the treatment through more frequent application.

Mild eczema is known to be more responsive to lower strength topical steroids. Results will show within the first few days, and often it comes with total clearance of eczema after one to two weeks of application.

On the other hand, the moderate cases of eczema may need more highly potent forms of topical steroids, which are often applied for at least two weeks before one can be able to observe improvements. For severe cases of eczema the use of topical steroids may only bring about partial improvements, even if treatment is extended to several months.

A general principle in treating atopic dermatitis with topical steroids is to use the least potent agent possible and limit the frequency of application. If the condition is severe and a more potent steroid is needed, the patient should be monitored closely, and the strength of the steroid should be reduced as the skin lesions improve.

TOPICAL IMMUNOMODULATORS. Another known treatment used for the treatment of eczema are topical immunomodulators, tacrolimus (Protopic®) and pimecrolimus (Elidel®) are calcineurin inhibitors approved by FDA (USA) for the treatment of atopic dermatitis. The topical immunomodulators have been demonstrated to be effective in the treatment of mild to moderately severe atopic eczema and have been shown to prevent any flare-ups when used as maintenance therapy.

Topical immunomodulators are effective as steroids pairing agents. When used in established eczema, their onset of action is generally slower compared to the topical corticosteroids, taking about three weeks to clear the eczema. The primary side effect when applied is the initial stinging sensation, or the general feeling of warmth or some mild itching. Topical immunomodulators do not cause skin thinning or adrenal suppression, which makes it principally useful for the treatment of eczema in areas that have thin skin such as the body folds, genital areas and the face.

ANTISEPTIC SOLUTIONS. Another well known solution are the antiseptic treatments can also be used in infected eczema as long as the formulation is not overly potent otherwise, these can have an abrasive and irritating adverse effect on the skin. Antiseptic bath oils are very useful in reducing the bacterial load in atopic dermatitis. Condy's crystals can be used only if it is prepared in a significantly weaker concentration. Other antiseptics such as cetrimide, dibromopropamidine, polynoxylin, chloroxylenol, povidone chlorhexidine iodine and triclosan can also be applied.

TAR PREPARATIONS. Tars and extracts of crude coal tar are often used to reduce the amount of topical steroids needed in chronic maintenance of eczema. Tar preparations have anti-inflammatory and antipruritic effects on the lesions of atopic dermatitis. These preparations are effective when used alone or with topical corticosteroids. Some tar preparations, especially gels, may contain alcohol and thus can be irritating. Shampoos, bath solutions and creams are less irritating. Tar preparations can be purchased over the counter.

The disadvantages of tars are, although it reduces itch and inflammation, they can be messy and often comes with an unpleasant smell and is known to be not as effective as topical steroids. Using the products at night and covering the treated areas can decrease these problems.

WET WRAPS. This therapy has proven effective in treating hand eczema and severe atopic dermatitis. Wet wraps are basically a form of a wet bandage that can be applied after the application of emollients or topical steroids. Wet-wrap therapy involves wrapping wet bandages around the affected skin. This is generally done before bedtime.

Wet wraps are used in acute cases of eczema with red, angry and highly inflamed conditions that may warrant the need for the patient to be admitted in the hospital. Wraps are able to rapidly gain control of the eczema. It primarily works with its moisturizing and cooling effect to the skin. They also provide skin protection from damage and scarring brought about by excessive scratching. Application can be administered for several days or possibly over an extended period. Wraps should also be reapplied as it gradually dries out.

With using wet-wrap, the skin gets re-hydrated, sleep will become more restful sleep, redness and inflammation is reduced, you will have less frequent itching and lesser possibility of finding Staphylococcus aureus (staph) bacteria on the skin.

ANTIBIOTICS

Atopic dermatitis reduces the skin's natural defenses, making it easier for skin to become infected. If a person's atopic dermatitis is not improving as expected, this may be because the skin is infected. Antibiotics are mostly used when there are symptoms of any form of bacterial infection, which is typically manifested by secretion of fluids and crusting, along with the observance of any pustules as well as the painful inflammation. This can be either orally or could be injected.

ORAL ANTIHISTAMINES

Severe itching can cause sleepless nights. In this case, doctors prescribe antihistamines to help reduce itch. This type of treatment is commonly used among children. The sedating antihistamines allow a better night's sleep for the child and his or her parents. Antihistamine creams should not be used on atopic dermatitis rashes because they contain chemicals that can actually worsen the rash.

PHOTOTHERAPY

Phototherapy or exposure to ultraviolet light may help adults with this condition. This treatment is rarely recommended for children because of its potential long-term side effects, including skin cancer and cataracts.

OTHER IMMUNE SUPPRESSING MEDICATIONS

There are ongoing investigations being undertaken to see whether these medications can treat atopic dermatitis. Most of them are used to treat other related diseases, such as psoriasis or allergic rhinitis. These medications include Cyclosporine, Interferon, Methotrexate and Azothiaprine. Also natural remedies can be applied to be able to treat atopic dermatitis. This include moisturizing your skin daily through proper ways of bathing and moisturizing and avoiding allergens such as dust, pollen, animal dander and certain foods that can cause allergic reaction. Also, keeping finger nails very short, smooth and clean can prevent damage from scratching especially when the itch is uncontrollable.

CONTACT DERMATITIS

Test is not a requirement for this condition because it is easy to recognize a contact allergy and no specific test can reliably show what the effect a substance will be to an individual case. However, patch tests may be used to determine whether the skin condition may be caused or aggravated by a contact allergy.

The rash associated with this condition usually (but not always) completely clears up if the allergen is no longer in contact with the skin, but recurs even with slight contact with it again. Treatment for contact dermatitis will depend on the cause and severity of the symptom as well as age and overall health. Treatments for this may include the following:

GENERAL AVOIDANCE OF THE IRRITANT

Contact dermatitis can be prevented by avoiding contact with the substance/s causing the irritation or allergy. Avoiding all substances that can trigger a flare-up can be difficult – and yet so impossible. If contact does occur, the material should be washed off immediately with mild soap and water or can be flushed off with water followed by the use of an antidote or specific remedy when toxic chemical or substance has burned the skin. During unavoidable circumstances, gloves and protective clothing may be helpful.

MEDICATIONS

Depending on the severity of the case, treatment with medications may also be an option. Such medications include:

CORTICOSTEROIDS. Corticosteroids are used in many inflammatory rashes. Applying a corticosteroid can help combat inflammation. This medication may be applied to your skin in a form of cream or ointment.

Corticosteroids or steroids are not related to the anabolic steroids that are misused by some athletes to increase performance. But for more severe cases, your healthcare provider may have to prescribe a stronger steroid medicine to be put on the affected area, taken by mouth, or given as an injection. One example of which is Prednisone that may be taken by mouth or injected.

ANTIHISTAMINES. Antihistamines, as mentioned earlier in atopic dermatitis, are used to control the itch. Prescription antihistamines may be given if nonprescription strengths are not adequate. Antihistamines may not be very effective but are sometimes taken at night if sleeping is a problem.

ANTIBIOTICS. When an infection develops at the site of contact dermatitis, antibiotics may be prescribed to treat the infection (usually flucloxacillin or erythromycin).

LOTIONS OR OTHER TREATMENTS

Shake lotions, such as calamine lotion and cool colloidal oatmeal baths may relieve itching and tend to be used for an extended period of time. As the name implies, shake lotions must be shaken before being applied in order to mix the active ingredient. When using sunscreens, those that do not contain PABA are the most recommended. Barrier cream such as those containing zinc oxide may help to protect the skin and retain moisture.

A mild bar soap or non-soap cleanser may also be recommended because normal soaps can dry the skin. When wearing jewelries made of nickel, cover them with a clear nail polish or special spay to prevent direct contact with the skin. And for best result, be sure to finish the recommended treatment program and all prescription medications.

DYSHIDROTIC DERMATITIS

Depending on how severe the condition is, individual treatment will vary. Most of the time no treatment is required and the rash or blisters will clear up on their own. The skin will take awhile to recover from this ailment and it can recur so you should be careful and take care of your skin. The following treatments have been used by Pompholyx sufferers. These are listed purely to show you that the symptoms can be addressed.

COOL COMPRESS

To relieve and dry up the blisters, soaks or compresses using weak solutions of Condy's crystals (potassium permanganate), aluminum acetate, or vinegar in water, can be applied for 15 minutes at four times a day. Compresses are not suitable for dry eczema.

EMOLLIENTS

Frequent rubbing of hand creams (emollients), dimeticone barrier cream for example, can keep the skin soft and however after application, the area must be kept dry.

TOPICAL STEROID

Potent topical steroids should be applied to the affected areas nightly. They help reduce inflammation and itching. The more potent products should not be used for more than two weeks unless your doctor advises otherwise. Steroid creams are used when the skin is blistered or weeping. Steroid ointments are used for the chronic dry stage.

ANTIBIOTICS

Antibiotics can be prescribed in this form of eczema in case secondary infection is present.

SYSTEMIC STEROIDS

Systemic corticosteroids are synthetic derivatives of the natural steroid, cortisol, which is produced by the adrenal glands. They are called "systemic" steroids if taken by mouth or given by injection as opposed to topical corticosteroids, which are applied directly to the skin.

The flares in this form of eczema might be quite explosive. In this case, doses of systemic steroids can calm down the flare and reduce the cause of an even large bulla and edema. But long term treatment with systemic steroids is rarely advisable because of the undesirable side effects.

PUVA THERAPY

PUVA means Psoralen & Ultra Violet 'A'. This kind of UV treatment is commonly administered to people with eczema, psoriasis and vitiligo, and mycosis fungicides. The PUVA therapy is a special type of UV treatment that involves soaking of the affected areas in psoralen solution and then exposing it to long waves of UV light.

This needs to be done frequently, sometimes even 4 to 5 times in a week and can last for many months. But it has been reported that smoking negatively influences the outcome of PUVA therapy in patients with dyshidrotic dermatitis.

NUMMULAR DERMATITIS

No treatment is uniformly effective but there are some that helps control or clear the nummular eczema. Even if the disorder is totally cleared, you will still be predisposed to have repeat episodes. Some treatments that can definitely help are as follows:

SUPPORTIVE CARE

Hand eczema may improve if vinyl gloves are worn at any time the hands come in contact with irritants. Rubber gloves should be avoided or worn over a pair of cotton gloves, as chemicals used in processing the rubber may aggravate the eczema or cause contact dermatitis. After washing, the hands should be thoroughly patted dry. Swelling of the legs may be controlled by wearing compression bandages or special stockings. In general, irritating fabrics (wool, silk, and rough synthetics) should be avoided. Absorbent, non-irritating fabric (cotton) should be worn next to the skin. Use lukewarm water, as hot water dries out the skin. When bathing, limit the use of soap to the face, armpits, genital area, and feet. It is possible to find a treatment routine that controls nummular eczema.

ANTIBIOTICS

Prescribed oral antibiotics may be given, along with use of tap water compresses, especially when weeping and pus in the affected areas are present. The antibiotics help fight any infection from developing since the rash can be susceptible to infection.

CORTICOSTEROIDS

Corticosteroid cream or ointment should be applied following a circular motion 3 times per day. An occlusive dressing is used to cover the treated skin, under a polyethylene film. Another option is to use a flurandrenolide- impregranted tape, which is generally best before bedtime.

Intralesional corticosteroid injections may be beneficial for the few lesions that do not respond to therapy. Occasionally, oral corticosteroids are required, but long-term use should be avoided.

ULTRAVIOLET LIGHT THERAPY

In more widespread, resistant, and recurrent cases, ultraviolet B radiation alone or oral Psoralen plus ultraviolet A or PUVA radiation may be helpful.

Repeat treatments may be needed and some individuals may require continuous therapy. Sometimes it can be helped by using moisturizers on a regular basis. Nummular Dermatitis may spread so it is important to control and limit its severity.

SEBORRHEIC DERMATITIS

Hygiene issues play a key role in controlling seborrheic dermatitis. Frequent cleansing with soap removes oils from affected areas and improves seborrhea. Patients should be counseled that good hygiene must be a lifelong commitment. Outdoor recreation, especially during summer, will also improve seborrhea, although caution should be taken to avoid sun damage.

The kind of treatment for patients with seborrheic dermatitis depends on its location on the body as well as the patient's age.

SEBORRHEIC DERMATITIS ON THE SCALP AND BEARD AREAS (Dandruff). For adults and adolescents, dandruff is effectively treated with a shampoo containing selenium sulfide or pyrithione zinc. Alternatively, ketoconazole shampoo may be used. The shampoo should be applied to the scalp and beard areas and left in place for five to 10 minutes before rinsing. This will give it time to work.

A moisturizing shampoo may be used afterward to prevent desiccation of the hair. After the disease is under control, the frequency of shampooing with medicated shampoos may be decreased to twice weekly or as needed. Topical terbinafine solution has also been shown to be effective in the treatment of scalp seborrhea.

For infants, a separate treatment should be undertaken. Seborrheic dermatitis in infants is commonly known as "cradle cap." Involvement may be extensive, but this disorder frequently clears spontaneously by six to 12 months of age and does not recur until the onset of puberty. Products to be used for treating this in babies are not as strong as those used in adults.

Start the therapy for infantile seborrheic dermatitis with frequent shampooing with a mild non-medicated shampoo. Brushing your baby's scalp with a soft brush, like a toothbrush, can help loosen scales or flakes. But be gentle when massaging or brushing your baby's scalp--a break in the skin makes it vulnerable to infection. If a non-medicated shampoo doesn't work, talk to your doctor about switching to a shampoo that contains tar.

Your doctor may recommend a prescription shampoo that contains ketoconazole. If scale is extensive in the scalp, the scale may be softened with oil, gently brushed free with a baby hairbrush and then washed clear.

SEBORRHEIC DERMATITIS ON THE FACE. Areas of the face affected by this form of eczema may be washed frequently with shampoos that are effective against seborrhea as mentioned above.

Alternatively, ketoconazole cream may be applied once or twice daily on the affected areas. Often hydrocortisone cream is added once or twice daily to affected areas to aid with resolution of erythema and itching. A lotion containing sodium sulfacetamide is also an effective topical agent for this.

For babies, gentle steroid lotions or creams may be used to treat seborrheic dermatitis.

SEBORRHEIC DERMATITIS ON THE BODY. Seborrhea of the trunk may be treated with frequent application of zinc or coal tar containing shampoos or by washing with zinc soaps. Additionally, topical ketoconazole cream and/or a topical corticosteroid cream, lotion or solution applied once or twice daily is proven to be very useful. Benzoyl peroxide washes are also helpful in controlling seborrhea of the trunk. Patients should be cautioned to rinse thoroughly after applying these agents as they will bleach clothing and bed linens. These agents may cause drying of the skin so patients may benefit from applying a moisturizer after every treatment. For severe seborrhea, unresponsiveness to the usual topical can be substituted with isotretinoin therapy. Treatment with daily doses of isotretinoin may result to improvement of severe seborrhea after four weeks of therapy. However, isotretinoin has potentially serious side effects and few patients with seborrhea are appropriate candidates for therapy. This agent must be used cautiously and only by physicians who are well versed in all of its adverse effects.

RECIPES

IF YOU SUFFER FROM ECZEMA, TRY THE FOLLOWING RECIPES

Healthy Skin Juice

Juicing is an important part of healing your skin. This highly alkalizing drink is designed to reduce inflammation, restore the acid-alkaline balance in the body and aid liver detoxification. Add parsley for extra body deodorizing benefits and fresh breath. Use these ingredients in any combination and in any amounts to suit your tastes.

Serves 2 or 2 days' supply for 1 adult, preparation time 5 minutes.

Serves 2 or 2 days' supply for 1 adult, preparation time 5 minutes.

Choose from the following:

• 4 stalks celery

• 2 peeled pears (must be ripe; avoid Asian/ Nashi or Ya pears) (s: the skin contains salicylates)

- 2 carrots, tops removed (s)

- 1/4 small beetroot (beet), scrubbed (s)

- 1 cup iceberg lettuce

- 1/2 cup red cabbage

- Handful of fresh parsley

- 1/2 cup fresh mung bean sprouts, rinsed

- Skin Friend AM (optional)

Wash and scrub the chosen vegetables and pears. Using a juicing machine, juice the fruits and vegetables, ending by adding a splash of filtered water.

Notes:

- Using a slow juicer retains more of the enzymes from the fruit and vegetables, but any type of juicer is better than none!

- If you are allergic to pears, use 1 red/golden delicious apple (contains medium salicylates — note all other apples contain high salicylates so should be avoided during the program).

Mung Bean Sprout Pancakes

Makes 6 small pancakes, preparation time 5 minutes, cooking time 15 minutes

- 200 g (7 oz) mung bean sprouts

- 3/4 cup filtered water or more for thinner consistency

- 1/2 teaspoon quality sea salt, or to taste

- 2 tablespoons arrowroot flour

- Parsley Oil (see below), for frying

Rinse the mung bean sprouts, drain well, then place into a blender with the water and salt. Blend on medium–high speed until it is almost a smooth consistency. The consistency should be that of a thin pancake so slowly add extra water until you reach this. Add the flour and blend again until smooth.

Place a frying pan over medium heat and drizzle in a little oil. When the pan is ready, add about 1 cup of the pancake mixture, swirling the pan slightly if you want thinner pancakes.

When browned on one side flip and cook until slightly brown on both sides. Repeat the process. Serve warm. Store leftovers in the refrigerator and reheat before serving.

Parsley Oil

Makes ½ a jar, preparation time 4 minutes

Parsley contains protective antioxidants that help to reduce the formation of glycation end-products, which can form when meats are cooked. Use this oil to baste chicken or lamb before roasting or grilling (broiling), or use it any time a recipe requires cooking oil.

• 2 teaspoons fresh parsley

• ½ cup rice bran oil (see notes)

Blanch the parsley in hot water for about 1 minute, then drain and dry with paper towels. Combine the parsley and oil in a high-powered blender until well blended. Then strain the oil using cheesecloth or muslin. Store in an airtight jar in the refrigerator and use within a couple of weeks.

Notes:

• If you are sensitive or allergic to rice or rice bran oil, use other low-salicylate oils such as sunflower oil or refined safflower oil.

• Important: check the oil does not contain artificial antioxidants such as E310–312, E319, E320 (BHA) and E321 (BHT) — they will make you itch like crazy.

Potato and Pesto Pizza

Serves 2, preparation time 20 minutes, cooking time 15 minutes

• 2–3 pieces Spelt Flat Bread (see below)

• 1 portion Parsley Pesto (see below)

- 3–4 white potatoes, peeled and finely sliced into discs

- Caramelized Leek Sauce (see below)

- quality sea salt, to taste

- 1/4 cup finely chopped fresh chives

- Handful of cashew nuts, chopped (optional)

Preheat the oven to 180°C (350°F). Insert a pizza stone into the oven before pre-heating or line a large flat baking tray with baking paper. Make the Spelt Flat Bread, Parsley Pesto and Caramelized Leek Sauce if not already prepared.

Place the flat breads onto the baking tray, spread with the pesto and add a thin layer of potato. Top with the leek sauce, adding dollops intermittently, and season with salt. Place the pizza in the oven and bake for about 15 minutes or until the potato is soft. Remove from the oven, top with chives and raw cashew nuts and serve.

Spelt Flat Bread

Makes 6, preparation time 10 minutes, cooking time 20 minutes

- 1 1/4 cups plain spelt flour, plus extra for kneading (wholemeal if available)

- 3/4 teaspoon finely ground quality sea salt

- 1 tablespoon Parsley Oil (see below)

- 2/3 cup boiling water

In a bowl, mix together the spelt flour and salt. Add the oil and hot water, and mix using a knife. The dough should not be sticky — if it is, add extra flour until it can be kneaded without sticking to the board.

Lightly flour your chopping board and turn out the dough onto the board. Knead the dough for approximately 3 minutes, until smooth and elastic (add more flour if dough is sticky), then cut into six balls of similar size. Add more flour to the chopping board, then flatten each ball with a rolling pin to make large, very thin circles — each flat bread should be about 20–22 cm (8–81 in) in diameter. You will need to add more flour as you go along to ensure the flat bread does not stick and can be rolled out paper-thin.

Heat a large non-stick frying pan over medium-high heat and cook each flat bread for about 1 minute each side, or until bubbles appear and the bread becomes browned in spots. For soft wraps, don't cook them for too long. The longer they are left in the pan, the crunchier they will be.

Caramelized Leek Sauce

Makes 4 servings, preparation time 5 minutes, cooking time 10 minutes

- 1 small leek, green part removed (about 2 cups chopped)

- 1 tablespoon Parsley Oil (see above)

- 2 tablespoons real maple syrup (adjust to taste)

- quality sea salt, to taste

Thoroughly wash the leek layers to ensure they are free of dirt. Finely chop the white parts and palest green parts of the leek. Heat the oil in a saucepan on medium heat and sauté the leek until very soft and slightly golden. Add the syrup and sea salt to taste and cook on low heat for another few minutes until sticky and golden.

FOODS TO EAT

For people with eczema, eating certain foods can trigger the body to release immune system compounds that cause inflammation, which, in turn, contributes to an eczema flare-up. An anti-eczema diet is similar to an anti-inflammatory diet.

Examples of anti-inflammatory foods include:

• Fish, a natural source of omega-3 fatty acids that can fight inflammation in the body. Examples of fish high in omega-3s include salmon, albacore tuna, mackerel, sardines, and herring.

• Foods high in probiotics, which are bacteria that promote good gut health. Examples include yogurt with live and active cultures, miso soup, and tempeh. Other fermented foods and drinks, such as kefir, kombucha, and sauerkraut, also contain probiotics.

• Foods high in inflammation-fighting flavonoids. Examples of these include colorful fruits and vegetables, such as apples, broccoli, cherries, spinach, and kale.

Eating more of these foods and cutting down on any trigger foods could help to reduce eczema flare-ups.

ELIMINATION DIET AND FOODS TO AVOID

Food-sensitive eczema reactions will typically occur about 6 to 24 hours after a person eats a particular food. Sometimes, these reactions may be delayed even longer.

To determine what foods may be causing the reaction, a doctor will often recommend an elimination diet. This diet involves avoiding some of the most common foods known to cause eczema.

Before eliminating any foods, a person will need to slowly add each food type into their diet and monitor their eczema for 4 to 6 weeks to determine if they are sensitive to any particular food.

If a person's symptoms get worse after adding a particular food to the diet, they may wish to consider avoiding it in the future. If a person's symptoms do not improve when eliminating a food, they probably do not need to remove it from their diet.

Some common foods that may trigger an eczema flare-up and could be removed from a diet include:

• Citrus fruits

• Dairy

- Eggs

- Gluten or wheat

- Soy

- Spices, such as vanilla, cloves, and cinnamonTrusted Source

- Tomatoes

- Some types of nuts

A doctor may also recommend allergy testing. Even if a person is not allergic to a particular food, they may have sensitivity to it and could experience skin symptoms after repeat exposure. Doctors call this reaction food responsive eczema.

People with dyshidrotic eczema, which typically affects the hands and feet, may experience benefits from eating foods that do not contain nickel. Nickel is found in trace amounts in the soil and can, therefore, be present in foods.

Foods that are high in nickel include:

- Beans

- Black tea

- Canned meats

- Chocolate

- Lentils

- Nuts

- Peas

- Seeds

- Shellfish

- Soybeans

Some people with eczema also have oral allergy syndrome or sensitivity to birch pollen. This means they may have reactions to other foods, including:

- Green apples

- Carrot

- Celery

- Hazelnuts

- Pears

People with eczema are more prone to oral allergy syndrome and should speak to their doctor if they have a pollen allergy or experience mild allergic reactions to the above foods.

DIETARY SUPPLEMENTS AND ECZEMA

Research has shown that taking probiotic supplements may reduce the symptoms of eczema. More studies are needed, however, to confirm the effectiveness and dosage required.

Probiotics are available in a variety of supplements, such as the selection available here. If a person is not sure which probiotics to buy, they may find the online reviews helpful and can also talk to their doctor.

Probiotics are also naturally present in many foods. Probiotic foods include:

• Yogurt

• Sauerkraut

• Kimchi

• Miso

• Tempeh

• Kombucha

Other supplements that have been studied trusted Source include fish oil and Chinese herbal preparations;

neither of which made a significant difference in eczema symptoms.

OUTLOOK

While a person's diet is not always a trigger for eczema, some people may find that their symptoms do get better when they make dietary changes.

Making these changes and monitoring the results can help a person determine whether changing their diet can help them better manage their condition.

If a person does eliminate a large food group, such as wheat-containing products, they may wish to talk to their doctor about supplements to ensure they are not missing out on any essential vitamins and minerals.

Why does eczema itch?

Eczema is a common skin disease that causes itchy, painful lesions that most people find challenging not to scratch. If a person scratches the skin eczema affects, it may thicken and become red and painful. Scratching can also lead to infection and scarring.

The National Eczema Association notes that the causes of eczema may have links to certain environmental triggers and genetics, although they are not sure of the exact causes of the disease.

Factors outside and inside the body trigger people with eczema's overactive immune systems, causing inflammation. The inflammation is responsible for the itchy rashes that people associate with eczema.

In this work, we examine why eczema itches and how to help prevent it. We also look at what happens to the skin when someone scratches their eczema and the possible treatment options.

Eczema itching triggers

Many environmental trigger factors may cause itching in eczema due to allergic reactions or irritants. These may include:

- Perfumes

- Soaps

- Pet dander

- Household cleaning products

- Detergents

- Synthetic and wool clothing

- Changes in temperature

- Contact allergy to latex, cement, or metal

- Dust

- Grass and trees

- Chemical substances

- Humidity

- Stress

- Cold and flu

- Certain foods

What happens when a person scratches eczema?

People experiencing a flare-up of eczema often experience an "itch-scratch cycle." This is when a person is itchy, and they scratch their eczema, which causes more inflammatory mediators to release, which in turn causes more itchy dry skin. The dry skin leads to more itching, and so the cycle continues.

Scratching, not eczema itself, is one of the main causes of skin damage. Scratching can lead to painful, red skin, which may break and bleed.

If a person's skin breaks, they are at higher risk for infection. Broken skin also makes it easier for irritants and allergens, such as dust and pet dander, to enter the skin barrier and cause eczema to flare.

Scratching can also cause the skin to become thick and leathery through a process called lichenification, which may cause changes to skin color. It may take weeks or months for the skin to return to its typical appearance.

Some people with eczema may have itchy lumps that may become thick and dark if they scratch them. This is called nodular prurigo. If this occurs in someone with a darker skin tone, there is an increased risk of the skin areas having permanent discoloration.

Scratching can also lead to scarring in the skin.

CONTACTING A DOCTOR

A person should contact a doctor or dermatologist about their eczema if:

• The lesions cover a substantial amount of the body

• It is affecting their daily living

• Over-the-counter products are not helping it

• The lesions have an infection, produce pus, and have red streaks.